Overcoming Emotional Burnout

A Practical Guide for Reclaiming Your Life

Allyson Hodge

Table of Contents

Introduction

Have you noticed that emotional burnout has become a widespread issue and talked about a lot? It is a state of overexertion and devastation that modern people face too often. Why does it happen? Daily life sped up and reached a pace that is not natural to human beings. However, we try hard to meet all of the demands and needs that appear out of nowhere all the time. We try to meet social expectations, to become successful, to gain wealth, build relationships, and be the best in all fields. In this book, we'll talk about emotional burnout— what it is, how it affects our lives, and, most of all, how to overcome it and prevent it from happening in the future.

Being emotionally burnt out feels like being emotionally drained. You feel exhausted and empty. Since there is not enough support availabe, you don't have a shoulder to cry on. You feel that you need to recharge emotionally, but it seems impossible since nothing brings you excitement or joy. You feel detached from everything and everyone.

Someone going through emotional burnout feels like they have nothing more to give. Their nervous system is exhausted from constant stress and they have no will or strength to cope with it anymore.

Everyday life seems like a constant demand to give more and more, which provokes even more stress. There doesn't have to be any particularly stressful situation. When you are emotionally burnt out, you feel like ordinary activities require too much of your emotional engagement and everything might be stressful.

A person who suffers from this condition feels no motivation or desire to take any action, even those that used to be pleasant. Everything seems too hard and brings no joy. Although they may seem to have everything put together, it's often thanks to a strong will to stay committed by sheer force.

Symptoms of emotional burnout may be very similar to certain clinical conditions, such as clinical depression. So it's important to visit a doctor to rule out depression. If depression is ruled out and a person is generally healthy, it may be a matter of emotional burnout. This is not an official mental health condition, but if not confronted, it might affect a person's health in more severe ways and provoke permanent damage. It's essential to take it seriously and cope with this condition in an efficient, proper way.

Emotional exhaustion might be a part of general burnout, or one may experience only emotional burnout. It happens due to accumulated stress from a situation in one's personal life. It could be related to any area: relationships, work, school, or any other aspect of one's life.

Anyone can experience emotional burnout, but people with demanding jobs or certain life situations are at high risk. People who are going through big life changes or grief are also at high risk, and the same goes for people with a chronic illness, financial issues or poverty, and people with demanding jobs such as caregivers, healthcare workers, police officers, firemen, teachers, even stay-at-home moms. The list is almost endless. Anybody facing constant and high stress is at risk for emotional burnout.

Effects of Not Dealing with Emotional Burnout

The fact that emotional burnout is not an official diagnosis may allow people to not take it seriously enough. You might think, "I'm just tired. I'll get over it after a short break or a vacation. It could also simply pass on its own." But it's not so simple. It's important to be aware of the effect of emotional burnout on mental and physical health if we do not deal with it. Below are some of the serious effects that emotional burnout may have on your health:

High levels of stress hormones. Stress hormones are crucial in helping us detect danger. They motivate us to take action to solve problems. When danger passes or a problem is resolved, the body goes back to normal. However, constant high levels of stress hormones are not healthy and their continuous release puts the body in a state of perpetually dealing with a threat. In other words, your heart is pumping faster, blood pressure is higher, blood sugar levels are increased, and the use of energy is higher than usual. The hormone called cortisol will take care to do what's most useful in a fight-or-flight mode, so it will affect your digestive system, reproductive system, and immunity.

Physical ailments. Since emotional burnout puts the body on the fight-or-flight mode, it can cause changes in sleeping patterns, eating habits, weight loss or weight gain, digestion problems, headaches, heart palpitations, and high blood pressure.

Problems in social interaction. Emotional burnout may also provoke problems in interactions within the family, with your loved ones, or co-workers. When you have to deal with difficult feelings like apathy, lack of motivation, anxiety, depression, low self-esteem, confusion, helplessness, and hopelessness, it might be difficult to maintain good communication with the people around you.

Those are just some of the issues you can expect if you don't find ways to deal with emotional exhaustion. Further, it may lead to more severe health issues and conditions, so one may develop depression or general anxiety disorder, heart disease, and other severe health problems that require serious treatment. Obviously, emotional burnout is a state that requires a serious approach and decisive action.

How to Recognize Emotional Burnout: Symptoms and Stages

If your doctor says everything's all right with your physical health and has also ruled out depression, but you still feel exhausted all the time and everything feels like a chore, you are probably in a state of emotional burnout.

Emotional burnout is manifested by many symptoms—physical, mental, and emotional. However, here are the main ones, categorized to make them easier to understand and recognize:

Physical Symptoms of Emotional Burnout

- Changes in sleeping patterns, sleeping problems, or insomnia
- Chronic lack of energy
- Frequent headaches
- Frequent colds and flus, weak immune system

Affective Symptoms of Emotional Burnout

- Lack of motivation
- Feeling anxious or depressed
- The feeling of failure, low self-esteem
- Feeling emotionally numb

- Absence of feeling joy, even while doing once enjoyable things
- Irritability
- Feelings of loneliness and detachment from the world
- Negative outlook and approach, pessimistic mood
- Lack of satisfaction

Behavioral Symptoms of Emotional Burnout

- Excessive use of food, alcohol, or drugs to cope
- Often snapping at people, demonstrating frustration to others
- Leaving tasks incomplete or avoiding work
- Procrastination or delaying things
- Isolating yourself from others at home or in the workplace
- Withdrawing yourself from responsibilities

If you recognize yourself among these symptoms, you are most likely going through emotional burnout. It's important to be aware of how you feel, to be honest with yourself, and to take your emotions and physical sensations seriously. They exist to guide you and to warn you if something's wrong. If you don't feel well, whether physically or emotionally, you need to do something about it.

Emotional burnout doesn't happen overnight. It's a gradual process and develops through stages. If you know about them, you'll be able to recognize even early symptoms and signs that you are tending towards a state of emotional exhaustion. This way, you'll be able to stop the process, reverse it, and avoid damage.

Four stages of emotional burnout

1) At the first stage, it might be difficult to recognize emotional exhaustion. In this phase, one is often still excited about a new job, new project, a new stage in life, or whatever the demanding situation is; or too occupied by grief, too busy to stop and ask themselves, "How am I?" A person feels tension. It can seem like positive tension, enthusiasm, or inspiration.

But the key point is that the person doesn't get enough rest. They are in constant motion, accumulating fatigue and stress. One is driven by high levels of stress hormones, and fatigue is often not recognized due to adrenaline rushes. When the person begins to notice high tension and stress, they tell themselves, "Be patient. You'll be able to rest soon. Hold on just for a while, you can catch a break when this is all over" and so on. But fatigue won't disappear and rest can't be postponed.

2) If the person ignores the growing tension and continues doing the same, the second stage of emotional burnout is inevitable. It's characterized by constant, extreme fatigue. One is able to hold everything together for a while, doing things automatically by mere inertia. At this stage, sleeping problems usually occur. One has trouble falling asleep or staying asleep during the night. A busy mind can't calm down enough to rest and recharge. And although it might seem like the person is getting enough sleep, they actually can't get enough rest because of the poor quality of sleep. After a few sleepless nights, it becomes harder and harder for them to remember their initial intention or purpose. The internal motivation and desire to achieve anything disappears and everything becomes just a list of chores that have to be done. It seems like everyone and everything requires more and more from you, but you feel drained as if there's nothing more to give. You are on the road to indifference.

3) Even feeling like this for many people is not enough reason for pressing pause. Those who are not aware of emotional burnout force themselves to go on with whatever is causing it. Their perspective changes and they truly believe that life has to be hard. Their negative outlook doesn't allow them to see any other possibility.

This all turns into irritability and even aggression. It might seem like you are lashing out at your kids, partner, or co-workers without an objective reason. Frequent outbursts of anger suggest that the tension has increased so much that the nervous system cannot cope. It needs to protect itself, so it reacts with bursts of anger.

However, lashing out and taking frustration out on others brings only temporary relief. After a person has an outburst, neither tension, nor fatigue, nor depression disappear. It's only replaced by exhaustion. The person might feel guilty for their behavior, but can't cope with it.

4) Your mind does almost everything it can to show you something's wrong. If you do nothing to help yourself, emotional burnout won't disappear. Eventually, it will turn into illness because the immune system can't protect you anymore from apathy or depression. At this level, you will have to face your issues but they will be far more severe than just emotional exhaustion.

Is emotional burnout related to stress?

Yes, but it's not the same as stress. Prolonged, poorly managed stress is one of the mechanisms of emotional burnout.

Constantly high levels of stress hormones drain you, leaving you burnt out emotionally. Engaging in prolonged stressful situations and going through major life changes like having a baby, going through a divorce, losing a loved one, or having a demanding job can make you chronically stressed and prone to emotional burnout.

However, not every aspect of stress is bad. Moreover, being stressed from time to time won't do you any harm. It can even have a positive impact on your nervous system and your performance. It can force you to put more effort into achieving your goals. When faced with stressful situations, the mind seeks ways to cope with it, and it activates internal resources, making you more active.

On the other hand, constant stress, like being endangered all the time, taking care of a newborn or an aging parent, doing a job you hate, or living with severe illness, doesn't give you any time to decompress or relax.

Five Channels for Overcoming Emotional Burnout

The first step in overcoming emotional burnout is realizing what's going on. A person needs to recognize and understand what is happening, and to accept this condition as reality. You are the only one responsible for your life, and the only person who can help you overcome this is you. Take some time to understand what's going on in your life and what is out of balance. Emotions are our primary system of navigation. If they show you something's wrong, trust them. You need to take care of your physical and mental well-being, and then the emotional level of your being will heal. It's crucial to admit how you feel and allow yourself to accept your emotions.

Once you do that, you can plan further actions for overcoming burnout. Your main internal compass should be adjusted to pleasure and relaxation. Activities that bring you joy will be your main source for recharging and curing emotional burnout.

Channels for facing emotional burnout head-on:

- Physical
- Mental
- Social
- Creative

- Affective

There are five channels that you can use to cope with emotional bunout: physical, mental, social, creative, and affective. The more of them you use, the sooner you'll manage to cope with the situation. In other words, you need to take care of your body and mind, to reexamine your belief system, connect with others, allow your creativity to express itself, and encourage and accept your emotions.

Taking Care of Your Body

Your body is the temple of your soul and the place where your emotions live. We are whole beings and there is a strong connection between our body, mind, and spirit. So it's crucial to take care of your body first so you can heal on all the levels. Begin with basics and give your body what it needs— proper rest, quality nutrients, hydration, and exercise. Further, you need to help it relax and recharge by doing pleasant and relaxing things that impact the senses, like massage, aromatherapy, spa treatments, and more.

Sleep

"Go get some sleep and everything will be fine" is not the ultimate advice for recovery, but there's a lot of truth to it. As with the whole body and mind, our emotions can't work well when we lack sleep. It's one of the most crucial ways to overcome emotional exhaustion. When you don't have the required seven to nine hours of sleep, many things change in your brain. One of them is that the amygdala, the part responsible for negative emotions and memories, works at full speed. On the other hand, the hippocampus, which should keep it in balance, is sleepy and can't function properly to balance your mood. So it's like driving a car at full speed without brakes. It's not surprising that you can't control your mood and that everything seems like a disaster. Lack of sleep contributes to feelings of sadness, anger, helplessness, hopelessness, pessimism, and a negative outlook. This won't help you at all if you are already emotionally exhausted.

Besides that, our whole body and mind suffers when we don't get enough sleep. The prefrontal cortex of the brain, the part responsible for our reasoning, planning, and memory, shrinks. If you don't let your body and mind sleep as much as they need, they don't get a chance to recharge, rejuvenate, and resolve small issues that surface during the day. Chronic lack of sleep can lead to many health issues and even shorten one's lifespan.

The first step in coping with emotional burnout is having a good night's rest. When you experience exhaustion, it's not unusual to suffer from insomnia and not be unable to shut down your busy mind. But don't let that get you down—you have to find ways to press pause.

Here is some advice on how to fall asleep easier and get some excellent, high quality healing slumber:

Decide it's time to recharge. Understand how vital sleep is for your mental health and emotional state, and how crucial its role is in overcoming emotional burnout. Set it as a priority and don't let anything else take its place. For instance, going to bed on time is more important than going out with friends, watching a movie, or even finishing a presentation for work tomorrow. Don't make compromises with your rest.

Set the proper sleeping environment. The bedroom should be reserved only for sleep and intimacy. Keep your working and sleeping spaces separated. This means no laptop in your bedroom. It should be a calming, clear, and airy space where you feel relaxed. When you enter the bedroom, you should leaving behind the outside world including work, worries, concerns, and duties.

The bedroom should be dark and well-ventilated. Our bodies need the dark to produce chemicals responsible for restoring our cells and maintaining optimal health. Turn off all the lights and dim the street lights with tick curtains, blinds, or use a sleeping mask. Let fresh air into the room a while before sleep. You'll fall asleep easier and sleep better. Also, take care that the temperature in the room is adequate. It should be around 64° F. Use heating or air conditioning to make sure it's not too cold or too warm.

Choose the right bedding. Comfortable mattress and pillows are must-haves for a quality night's sleep. So choose as high quality as your budget allows. When it is about bedsheets and covers, choose natural materials such as cotton.

Create an evening routine. Our minds love routine. It lets you always know what you're doing before bed without wasting energy on planning and thinking about it. Your mind knows what's coming, in which order, and feels calm and safe. When the evening routine becomes a signal for your brain that it is time for sleep, it can easily switch into preparing for sleep. Your evening routine should be relaxing, so it should consist of everything you need to do before bed, from brushing your teeth and showering, to a cup of tea, to guided meditation. Choose whatever works for you, as long as it has a soothing effect.

Go to bed early at the same time every night. It's scientifically proven that sleep before midnight is far more effective than sleep after midnight. Some hormones, like melatonin, are produced only during the first half of the night. Try to go to bed before 10:00 p.m. and stick to your bedtime, even over weekends. It might sound like a loss, but it will pay off because it plays a significant role in coping with emotional burnout. The first time you wake up full of energy, reborn, you'll understand the value of this advice.

Calm down before going to bed. This one is simple. You have to slow down and be calm in order to fall asleep. If you don't, it will take you more time to fall asleep. Instead of enjoying a pleasant bedtime routine and going to bed early, you will be lying there, staring at the ceiling, with your mind rushing in all directions until past midnight.

If you don't have a habit of calming down before sleep, here are some ideas on what to include in your evening routine:

Unplug. Turn off all ringers, notifications, and screens. Whatever you watch or read before sleep, you are taking with you into sleep. And you don't need excess pieces of information for your mind to process. Blue light from screens has the effect of stimulating your brain, which is the opposite of what you are trying to achieve.

Dim lighting. The invention of artificial light is what has most interfered with our natural circadian rhythm. Bright light, artificial or not, tells your mind it is time to wake up. Dim light calms your nervous system, preparing it for the night's rest. Spend hours just before sleep in a softly lighted space.

Choose calming activities like reading, listening to soothing music, meditation, lighting candles, having a bubble bath, or drinking a calming tea.

Use lavender oil. The lavender scent is excellent for aiding relaxation and sleep. You can use it as an essential oil in your bath, spraying it on your pillow, or lighting a scented candle with lavender fragrance.

Try guided sleep meditation. Meditation is an excellent way to relax before sleep. You only need to get comfortable and listen to the voice of a narrator that guides you through a restful meditation. It will help you relax your whole body and fall into a deep, energizing sleep.

Choose the right bedtime tea. Sipping a cup of warm herbal tea has a soothing effect. Some of the best-known are chamomile, valerian, lavender, lemon balm, and spearmint or combinations of those ingredients. Bedtime teas combine anti-anxiety and pro-sleep herbal ingredients, helping to create a relaxing bedtime experience that reduces stress and anxiety. The sedative effect of these teas is mild, but the ritual of drinking a cup of tea is calming enough to help you fall asleep.

Breathing

Breathing is the simplest yet one of the most powerful ways to relax your body and mind.

However, we are often not even aware of how we do it.

Pay attention to your breathing. Notice any movement in your body connected to breathing. Does your stomach expand as you exhale or does the air fill only your chest? Breathing right is a precious skill we all knew as children, but over time, we forget and start to breathe shallowly, filling only our lungs instead of breathing deeply from the diaphragm and belly. Shallow breathing activates your sympathetic nervous system and triggers fight-or-flight mode, keeping you switched on to stress all the time. Deep, slow breathing does the opposite, calming you down.

Learning to breathe deeply can solve many of your issues, including exhaustion. You can use intentional, relaxed breathing to remain calm, grounded, support your health, and help yourself overcome emotional burnout.

Like every other skill, deep breathing requires practice. There are numerous breathing techniques, but try to do it at least three times a day in five-minute chunks. Ideally, you should take six breaths a minute. If you can't reach this number, don't stress over it. Do the best you can.

Here's how to do this breathing exercise. Find a comfortable place and sit upright with your spine straight. Make sure that all restrictive clothing and belts are loosened. Take a deep breath in through your nose so that your stomach expands. Fill your stomach and then your chest, counting to five. Breathe out slowly through your nose to the count of six. Feel your stomach shrink as you exhale. Set an alarm to go off so you can focus only on this exercise for a full five minutes, three times a day.

This exercise will help you to relax and boost your energy levels, but also over time and with everyday use, it will help you overcome emotional burnout and prevent it from happening in the future.

Food for overcoming emotional burnout

When we go through an emotionally exhausting period, we often neglect our basic needs. When you don't take care of your diet and eat junk food to gain energy to cope, your body and mind remain undernourished and suffer. You feel too exhausted to take care of your diet and that contributes to further exhaustion, becoming a vicious cycle. Although it might seem that your emotional exhaustion has nothing to do with food, you need to clean up your diet to gain energy and overcome this condition.

What to avoid

Caffeine, alcohol, tobacco, drugs. When you are trying to overcome emotional burnout, what you need most is calmness and tranquility. Although a favorite drink of many, coffee is not the best choice when you are burnt out. Caffeine has a stimulative effect on body and mind. It may increase anxiety or a depressed mood, and masks tiredness, enabling you to use more energy than you actually have. It may also interfere with sleep. Be careful and find your ideal intake for caffeine—it might be one or two cups a day, or no coffee at all. When it comes to alcohol, tobacco, and drugs, there's not even one good reason to use them. Make your health a priority and cut them out of your diet completely.

Refined sugar. Even though we are used to consuming sweets, refined sugar will never be good for our health. It's most apparent when you suffer from adrenaline and sugar peaks and crashes. Eating dessert seems like a good idea when you lack energy, but the effects are short-term. Soon, the level of sugar in your blood drops, leaving you even more exhausted than before. Try to switch refined sugar with natural sweets like honey and nuts, or drink lemon water instead. When you feel a craving for sweets, first ask yourself if you are thirsty or tired and actually need water or a short nap.

Processed food. When it's about nutrition, quick solutions are the worst. If you eat junk food, fast food, food enriched with salt and sugar, and packed in tons of plastic, your body receives calories, but lacks needed nutrients. It doesn't get the required vitamins, minerals, or protein. Try to cut out processed food and focus on healthy eating and home cooking instead.

Inflammatory food. When you want to achieve mental and emotional balance, you need your body to be balanced as well and not provoke mood swings. That's why it would be wise to check if you are intolerant to gluten or dairy. Those foods may create allergic reactions and trigger mood changes in many people without them even realizing it.

What to include in your diet:

Whole foods, fruit, veggies, soups, and smoothies. Eating only foods that are not processed and packed in layers of plastic is natural. When you change your diet for this kind of food, you'll have more energy to cope with emotional burnout. When you feel strong and refreshed, it's easier to recover your normal emotional balance.

Include more veggies and fresh fruit, natural oils, nuts and seeds, eggs, fish, organic meat, and whole grains in your diet. Soups and smoothies are excellent ways of consuming a lot of nutrients, healthy fats, fiber, and antioxidants that you wouldn't normally get. You can add different supplements and healthy ingredients to boost the nutritive value of smoothies and soups. Make sure that you're fueling your body with meals prepared at home. It's the healthiest way, and cooking is a relaxing, calming activity for a busy, exhausted mind.

Omega-3 fatty acids. Ingesting enough healthy fats is essential since the human body needs them. Omega-3 fatty acids are known for increasing mood and soothing symptoms of anxiety and depression. Healthy fats also help us to absorb vitamins and antioxidants more efficiently. Try to include healthy fish in your menu at least three times a week.

Supplements. Some ingredients we need to boost our mental health are not contained in our usual diet in enough amounts. When we are stressed, our body spends all the reserves of certain vital chemicals. That's why it might be great to take them as supplements. Although it is not therapy, some additional nutrients like magnesium can work miracles for your mental balance and help you recover from emotional burnout. Four to six weeks are usually enough for you to start seeing positive effects. You might try some vitamin and mineral complexes that contain combinations of magnesium bis-glycinate, zinc, vitamin C, omega 3, B vitamin complex, electrolytes, holy basil, flaxseed oil, or licorice root extract.

Drink more water. It's surprising how much we forget to drink enough water, especially when we are exhausted. We tend to drink a lot of coffee to gain energy to keep up, but caffeine is a diuretic and can't be a substitute for water. It does the opposite, contributing to dehydration. It would be ideal to drink eight 8 oz. glasses of water a day. Follow your thirst, it's a perfect sign that you need water. The color of your urine is a good indication if you're getting enough. Its color should be a very light yellow if you're getting enough. For tastier water, add some lemon, mint, other fruit, or berries.

How to organize healthy eating

When you are already drained, it may seem like a mission impossible to put so much attention and effort into your diet. It's far easier to keep old bad habits and just grab something on the go. But if you want to help yourself overcome the condition you're in, you need to change your habits. Your body is one of the channels you need to use to recover, and healthy eating is one of the crucial things that require your attention. Don't give up on a healthy diet. Instead, make a good and sustainable plan.

Plan your meals in advance. Ideally, make a weekly menu and a grocery list for the whole week. Then stock up on healthy foods and you'll have everything you need for sticking to your new eating habit. If you don't have a plan or stock up on healthy food, you'll easily slip back into eating junk food.

Eat more small meals instead of large ones. Oscillation of sugar levels is unpleasant for both your mood and health. It's the last thing you need when trying to overcome emotional burnout. Rather than having two large meals a day, it's a better idea to divide them into smaller portions throughout the whole day. If your body doesn't feel good, don't give it more trouble by skipping meals or reducing your calorie intake.

Workouts for overcoming emotional burnout

When we are constantly busy and stressed, we neglect all our needs, including exercise. It seems like a natural way to save energy; our body doesn't want to waste energy while it's struggling to survive all that stress. But when you want to overcome the condition of emotional exhaustion, a workout will help you tremendously. It helps by getting you out of your head and into your body and physical effort. Movement improves your outlook by producing mood-elevating hormones and neurotransmitters like serotonin, dopamine, and endorphins. Exercise has antistress effects and breaks down stress hormones, helping you to relax. Finally, workouts strengthen your body, helping you cope with burnout.

If you're going through emotional burnout, a hard workout is not recommended. All activities, including exercise, should be moderate and oriented to joy and relaxation. Find out what kind of movement is joyful for you. You don't just need a workout routine that will strengthen your body, but one that will be enjoyable. Some recommended physical activities include walking, yoga, and swimming.

Walking, especially in nature, is underestimated in the modern world, while the negative consequences of our sedentary lifestyle are growing. Walking might be the best way to exercise when you are going through emotional burnout. It helps to clear your head, relax, improve breathing, and boosting metabolism without exhausting an already tired body and mind. You may combine it with socializing by walking with friends or by being surrounded by the healing power of nature. Choose a pleasant route and take your dog with you if you have one—there's no better company for cheering yourself up. After a good walk, you'll fall asleep easier, have better quality sleep, and feel more energized in general.

Another great way to exercise while being emotionally burnt out is practicing yoga. If you already have some experience with yoga, you can do it by yourself. Otherwise, find a yoga teacher. Yoga is not just about movement. It brings your body, mind, and spirit back into balance. According to yoga teaching, when you are out of balance, your chakras (energy centers) and nadis (energy channels) may be over or under-stimulated. This inhibits or poorly directs prana's flow (energy or life force) and can cause a sense of feeling stuck or stagnant. Practicing yoga will help you find equilibrium again. Yoga will help you exchange confusion for clarity, quiet the mind, and find inner peace. Besides that, your body will thank you for such quality training of stability, flexibility, and strength.

Swimming is also a great choice and not only during hot summer months. Combining the relaxing effects of water and movement, it's a gentle yet powerful workout for exhausted individuals. Spending time in the water will make you feel refreshed and as if all of your hard thoughts and feelings are being washed away.

Body relaxation

Another great way to improve your emotional state using the physical channel is to relax your body. Body and mind are connected on many levels and they affect each other. When your mind is busy, worried, and exhausted, your body is tense too. But if you manage to relax your body in spite of this, your mind will become more calm. When you focus on physical sensations, similar to while working out, you move your focus away from disturbing thoughts and allow your mind to rest.

There are many ways to relax your body and it should become a daily practice of recharging, not just as an aid in case of emotional burnout. Some of the most common means of relaxation are meditation, massage, and spa treatments.

Meditation

Meditation is well-known as a powerful means of relaxation. If you haven't tried it yet, now is the time. It will help you combat emotional exhaustion through reconnecting with your body, experiencing a sense of flow, being grounded and consciously present, and calming your mind.

To get started, try out some of the guided meditations for relaxation on YouTube. All you need is some quiet time alone. It's enough to do it just ten minutes a day to begin to experience benefits. Soothing meditations are focused on relaxing the whole body, part by part, and on breathing.

You can try it even without a guided program. Find a comfortable place. Sit or lie down, whatever is more convenient. Observe your breathing. No need to change anything, just notice your breathing—if it's fast and shallow or slow and deep. Notice any movement in the body connected with your breath. Try to focus on the physical sensations it provokes.

Move your attention to your toes and feet. Relax them. Then move your awareness up to your lower legs. Allow them to relax completely. Focus upward and relax your thighs, hips, pelvic area, and glutes. Feel the sense of complete relaxation in the whole lower half of your body.

Feel the life in your fingers. Allow your fingers and palms to relax, open them towards the ceiling. Relax your wrists and lower arms. Moving upward, relax your elbows and upper arms.

Bring your attention to your stomach. Notice how it is moving in the rhythm of your breathing. Relax it completely. Take another deep breath and fill your chest with air. Exhaling, allow your chest and ribcage to relax completely.

Focus on your back now. Feel the surface behind it. Imagine your spine relaxing and your vertebra in perfect alignment. Relax the whole back from the lowest point and upward, part by part. Feel all those heavy back muscles relax, becoming loose and elastic.

Take a deep breath and when you exhale relax your shoulders. Shoulders are the most important part of relaxation. Allow them to loosen and drop down from your ears. Relax your neck and throat. Allow your head to sink deeper onto the surface. Relax your scalp, your ears, and your forehead. Relax your facial muscles. Allow your jaw to release. Relax your chin, your lips, and the base of your tongue. Relax your cheeks and eyebrows. Relax the tiny muscles around your eyes and allow your eyes to rest completely.

Now your entire body is relaxed. Enjoy this feeling. Feel like you're floating while being supported. Feel the comfort and peace. Focus on your breathing, breathe deeply and slowly, inhaling through your nose, and exhaling slowly through your mouth. Allow your mind to rest and calm down, bringing your attention back to your breathing whenever your mind starts to wander. You are in a state of deep relaxation now. You can do this whenever you need to release tension. It will help you tremendously to recharge and recover from emotional burnout.

Relaxing massage and spa treatments

The mechanism that a massage helps you relax is the same one that works during meditation or a workout, bringing your focus to physical sensations, to the present moment, and relaxing the body.

Try out different types of massage until you find out which one suits you the most. There are numerous variations from hand massage with aromatic oils to massage with volcanic stones. Combining relaxing touch, scents of aromatic oils, soothing music, and a calming atmosphere, relaxing massage is a unique experience that can go a long way towards overcoming emotional burnout. By treating and pampering your body this way, you are showing self-love and creating a secure environment for your emotional being to heal.

Going to a spa is also a popular and beloved way to relax and de-stress. There are very few things more luxurious than pampering yourself with spa treatments. Visiting a spa is a great opportunity to have some me-time and separate yourself from everyday worries and sources of stress. This is time for you to relax and wind down, but the benefits of visiting a spa last longer than your appointment. You'll feel great after you leave, too.

One of many benefits of spa treatments is that they have an effect on your happiness levels. During the treatments and massage, your body releases serotonin, a hormone responsible for the feeling of happiness. It improves your mood during and after the visit, so you will experience a boost in your mood in the subsequent days as well.

Among their many benefits, spa treatments and massage improve sleep quality, helping you to catch more precious z's, which is extremely helpful if you already have sleeping issues due to emotional burnout. Being exhausted, you might be suffering from frequent headaches and other pains. Spa treatments and massage help to reduce those, too. Their benefits extend far beyond the massage table.

Taking Care of Your Mind

Rethink your system of beliefs, values, and goals

Our belief system consists of everything we genuinely believe about the world, ourselves, and how life should be. Its formation begins when we are very young and don't have the ability to form our own opinions, but we learn them from our loved ones. The problem is, our beliefs often don't support us or who we are. This is why we need to rethink them.

If you believe you have to do certain things a certain way or believe that you are responsible for others' happiness or you don't believe you deserve to be gentle with yourself, your behavior will inevitably lead to emotional burnout.

Think about why you are going through this. What brought you here? Which of your beliefs are connected to it? For instance, you might believe a man has to be successful at work at any cost, even neglecting his family. And now your belief is not in alignment with your feelings, making you exhausted. Or if you are a stay-at-home mom of young children, you might believe you have to do everything on your own, to be a super-mom. You need to reexamine the beliefs that brought you here.

Think about your values. Do you know what they are? Perhaps they are health, family, finances, love. They all need your attention and they are all significant. But if you value your finances, for instance, over your health or family, soon or later you'll have problems in those two areas. You need to define your priorities and each one should have its own place.

Ask yourself what your goals are. Define them and think about your purpose and what you have to offer to the world. Think about how to incorporate all of that into your everyday life so that your actions, thoughts, and emotions are in alignment. If any of your goals require neglecting some important value in your life, like health or family, seriously consider if it is worth so high a price. Everything you do needs to be in alignment with your values.

Adopt a positive mindset

Your life reflects the way you think—you probably already know that. But although you might know how beneficial it is to be a positive thinker, it might be challenging when you are emotionally exhausted. When you are sleep deprived, your amygdala, the part of the brain responsible for emotional regulation, goes into overdrive. It seems almost impossible to think positively. But it is achievable and just requires some effort. Positive thinking is a habit and a skill. It can be learned and practiced. Moreover, it demands daily practice if you want to switch entirely to a positive way of thinking and embody optimism. Although it might be hard, now is the time. It will help you combat and avoid emotional burnout.

Start small. Try to find the good in everything: all the people you meet, all situations. No matter how small, there are always some positive aspects. Think about things you can be grateful for—things that many of us take for granted. Start with your body and its incredible function, your home and everything within it, people who make your life better, activities you enjoy, anything that brings you comfort or joy.

Try to start your mornings with thoughts of gratitude and finish your days with those kinds of thoughts. You can even start a gratitude journal. Allow yourself to daydream and visualize everything you want to have or achieve in your life. Imagine things the way you want them to be.

Put an end to negative talk. This includes both self-talk and conversations with others. Stop complaining for good. You always have a choice about what you talk about. Decide to think, read, listen to, and talk only about positive things. Be sure that everything you discuss is true, useful, and awakens positive emotions in you and the people you talk to.

Be careful about the content you take in. Your mind is feeding on it, so be cautious about what you are reading on social media, listening to in the news, and every other source of information you consume.

Positive thinking is a daily practice. It has to be trained every day, like our muscles. Use affirmations to build positive beliefs. You can find numerous methods and techniques for adopting and developing a positive way of thinking. This will make you more relaxed, improve your mood, and make you more resilient to stress and emotional exhaustion.

Socializing

We are social beings, which means that connections with others are the heart of our well-being. It's scientifically proven that the main difference between happy people and those who are not, and also between people with long lifespans and those who live fewer years, is in the quality of their personal relationships. In other words, growing and maintaining your positive connections and relationships are your ticket for a joyful and long life. All the relationships you have in your life count—your partner, family, friends, and colleagues.

It's important to realize that social connection is one of the channels to heal from emotional burnout. It might be hard to reach out to others when you feel emotionally exhausted and drained. But it's crucial to do it and it will help you immesurably. Your loved ones will be glad that you show initiative. Include time with your family and friends into your schedule and commit to doing it, even when you don't feel like it. Talk to your trusted friends or family members and let them know what you are going through. They might have some piece of advice or cheer you up. It might just be enough for you to know that someone cares about how you feel and that they are there for you. Everything is much easier when you have support.

Customize social activities so they can fit into your recovery process. For instance, if it's too exhausting to go out to a club, go for a walk or have a healthy drink in a cafe with your best friend. Maybe you are not in a mood for a big family event, but you can spend some time playing with kids. If you are not the best company for a shopping tour, you might find it more pleasant to sip tea and chat with a friend.

Spending time with your close friends and family will make you feel comforted, cared for, less tense, and stronger in facing anything. Serving others, engaging in fun or humanitarian activities, will bring you a sense of meaning and satisfaction. Even small things like random acts of kindness can make you feel great. When trying to overcome emotional burnout, it's crucial to feel good as much and as often as you can.

Don't hesitate to seek help

If you are emotionally exhausted, you most likely need help. It is not a sign of weakness; it is human. No one should have to carry everything on their shoulders. Perhaps you believe that you need to do everything on your own, but it's time to change this.

You need to ask for support, reach out for help, delegate, and share work.

Include your close friends and family in what's going on. They will probably be glad to help. If they don't know you're struggling, it's not surprising they think you don't need support. Don't shy away from asking for help. Connect with new people and reconnect with those you already have in your life. Be sincere. It is not a sign of weakness to say you're struggling with emotional burnout. It just means that you've carried too much on your back. Social connections are a powerful aid against bad moods, anxiety, depression, and burnout. Life is simply much better with dear people to rely on.

Besides surrounding yourself with your loved ones, you might need professional help too.

To start healing, visit your physician to rule out everything else in order to conclude you are just emotionally drained. They might suggest different types of testing. Besides that, since emotional burnout is not an official medical condition, you might want to see different types of healers. There are psychologists, psychotherapists, naturopaths, acupuncturists, massage therapists, nutritionists, yoga teachers, and homeopathy healers. There are many professionals who can help you overcome this condition. You just need to find one whose approach suits you the best.

Pick which paths work best for you and make your own plan to overcome emotional burnout. For instance, you might want to see a psychotherapist, get a diet plan from a nutritionist, go to yoga classes, and follow a motivational speaker on YouTube. This book may also be your best friend on this journey.

Creativity, Laughter, and Play

Modern society appreciates seriousness, being constantly busy, a lack of "idle" time, and full use of energy. On the other hand, being relaxed, optimistic, cheerful, and smiling is often labeled as immature or silly. Through education we are taught to laugh less, to be more serious, to be less creative, to absorb information, to stop playing, and do "productive" things instead. It's not surprising that as grown-ups we forget to play, to laugh, and be creative. But when you only do serious things all the time, life isn't fun at all. You'll soon become emotionally and physically drained, burnt out, and have no will to get out of bed.

Emotional burnout is a sure sign that this is what has happened to you. It's time to bring those precious things to your everyday life again.

When it comes to creativity, you don't have to be Da Vinci to allow yourself to create. Try to remind yourself of what you loved to do as a kid. It might be drawing, painting, creating things, decorating, singing, dancing. Whatever it used to be, why not start to do it again and see if it still brings you joy? You can also find new hobbies, maybe sewing, pottery, playing guitar, whatever you like. Spend time on searching and trying out different things until you find out which you enjoy the most. Then make some time in your schedule for that activity on a daily or weekly basis.

When you do something you enjoy, it helps you focus, grounds you in the present, makes you immediately happier, and absorbs your attention. When you lose yourself in reading, for example, the outside world disappears. And that is exactly what you need—to disconnect from the outside world for a time and recharge your batteries with positive energy.

Make room for play and laughter

Living without play and laughter is not fun at all. It's not surprising if you feel empty and lifeless. Bring joy, play, and laughter back into your life. Turn your priorities upside down and make joy the top priority. There's nothing that laughter can't ease or make less hard. However, this is something we lose somewhere along the way. Over time, everything starts to seem so serious and black and white.

Decide to rediscover laughter, play, and joy, even if you've forgotten how. You can experience them again. Allow yourself free time for whatever makes your soul dance. Watch funny videos or a comedy, read books, hang out with friends, listen to music, dance, go for a walk, a run, a swim. Create whatever you like, bake cookies, construct model airplanes, draw maps of hidden treasure, grow bonsai... It doesn't matter what you choose as long as it makes you feel great. Feed your soul and tickle your funny bone. This is the sure way out of emptiness and emotional burnout.

Emotions

The connection between emotions and emotional burnout is obvious, yet not so simple to parse. Emotions are our main tool of navigation. You became exhausted because you didn't pay attention to yours and suppressed them for a long time. Now you might feel empty, as if all feeling has disappeared. However, your feelings are one of the channels that can get you out of this condition. How?

First, it might seem like there are no emotions at all. But as you start to take care of your physical and mental health, and use social and creativite channels for recovery, your feelings will begin to surface. Your task is to notice, observe, and accept them, no matter what. Denying, ignoring, and suppressing them is what brought you here. In order to move on, you have to do the opposite.

Allow yourself to feel all emotions—positive and negative. Don't force yourself to be constantly positive at any cost. Let yourself experience them all, but don't wallow for too long with depressing ones. Allow them to drift away and find ways to bring yourself into balance.

Positive emotions—joy above all the others— should be your guide. Try to choose thoughts that make you feel good, energized, motivated, and optimistic. Choose enjoyable activities. Choose the company of people who make you laugh and feel grateful to have them in your life. You always have the ability to choose. Always pick pleasant options that bring you joy. Doing so day by day and developing a positive mindset will allow your life to become magnificent, vibrant, and colorful again.

How to Prevent Emotional Burnout in the Future

To prevent emotional burnout, it is important to use all of the channels possible for feeling balanced. In short, you need to work on your inner peace, rest enough, take care of your diet and exercise, delegate certain responsibilities, preserve your relationships, express yourself creatively, and stay connected to your emotions.

Take care of your mental balance. Don't allow yourself to neglect your mental hygiene ever again. It's something that requires action on a daily basis. It doesn't have to take much time—10 minutes a day is enough for meditating or journaling. Small steps will keep you in good mental shape.

Get enough rest. Sleep should not be a cure for being emotionally drained. It is a basic human need. Let a healing eight-hour sleep become the norm, not an emergency aid for combating serious exhaustion. It's also not enough to have two weeks of vacation once a year. Everybody needs daily, weekly, and annual rest to recharge, far from stressors. To prevent yourself from burning out again, make quality night sleep a priority, with no excuses.

Treat yourself with love. You can't sip from an empty cup. In other words, you have to take care of yourself first so you can function and help others. Taking care of yourself is not selfish; it's a necessity. Be gentle. Afford yourself enough rest, a nourishing diet, enough pleasant movement, plenty of water, and deep breathing. Treat yourself with massages and spa visits, relaxation, taking a nap, eating a fruit salad, whatever makes you feel pampered and cared for.

Delegate. You don't have to and should not do everything on your own. Share obligations and tasks with your family and colleagues instead of pushing yourself to the edge of exhaustion.

Socialize. Connections and relationships with our friends and family determine our level of happiness. We are also more likely to fall into emotional burnout if we feel lonely. Reach out to people, make connections, and cultivate them so you can build your supportive network. Positive interactions will significantly enrich your life and prevent future emotional exhaustion.

Find your creative outlet. Creativity lowers stress levels and increases feelings of joy. It also strengthens connections with your emotions. No matter what type of creative activity you choose, it will keep you engaged and motivated. So revive an old hobby or find a new way of expressing yourself. It might be through colors, sound, movement, whatever makes you feel amused and entertained, allowing you to express your creative side.

Follow your heart and develop a positive mindset. Becoming resilient to stress is the best protection and prevention against emotional exhaustion. Start working towards adopting a positive mindset. Each day notice all of the good things you can be appreciative of. Practice the attitude of gratitude and take care of your mental hygiene on a daily basis. Do your best to feel good as often as possible, but allow yourself to experience and accept all of your emotions. Don't underestimate their importance. Trust them, since your feelings are your best system of navigation through life.

Printed in Great Britain
by Amazon

54898725R00033